MY FOOD
JOURNAL

*A Daily Companion
for Weight Loss
& Better Health*

KASEY HORN

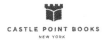

CASTLE POINT BOOKS

NEW YORK

MY FOOD JOURNAL. Copyright © 2019 by St. Martin's Press.
All rights reserved. Printed in Turkey.
For information, address St. Martin's Press,
120 Broadway, New York, NY 10271.

www.castlepointbooks.com

The Castle Point Books trademark is owned
by Castle Point Publishing, LLC.
Castle Point books are published and distributed
by St. Martin's Press.

ISBN 978-1-250-25306-4 (trade paperback)

Design by Joanna Williams

Our books may be purchased in bulk for promotional,
educational, or business use. Please contact your local
bookseller or the Macmillan Corporate and Premium
Sales Department at 1-800-221-7945, extension 5442,
or by email at MacmillanSpecialMarkets@macmillan.com.

First Edition: December 2019

10 9 8 7 6 5 4 3 2 1

Today is the day I start making real progress toward

(Fill in your goals.)

Whether your goals include losing weight or simply eating healthier, this journal can help you achieve them! The easy-to-use log pages that follow help you capture your daily food choices, key nutrition information, and calorie-burning activities in an attractive, portable book. Journaling powers weight loss and better health in two ways:

◆ First, the simple act of recording holds you accountable and inspires you to give more thought to the food and activity choices you make.

◆ Second, seeing your choices all together in a quick-to-review format helps you spot what's working and moving you toward your goals and what could be holding you back. In fact, there's space at the end of each log to rate the day and note what went well and what needs more attention.

Just a few minutes spent at each meal and snack time will help you stay on track and fuel your mind, body, and spirit with the healthy choices you deserve. With 192 pages, this book provides plenty of space to follow through with your journaling habit for more than 90 days. When you reach the last journaling page, look back and celebrate your successes— and treat yourself to a new journal to continue on your healthy track!

DATE: / /

Mon ● Tue ● **Wed ●**
Thu ● Fri ● Sat ● Sun ●

BREAKFAST	Time:	Amount	Calories	Protein	Carbs	Fat	
Breakfast Totals							

SNACK	Time:	Amount	Calories	Protein	Carbs	Fat	
Snack Totals							

LUNCH	Time:	Amount	Calories	Protein	Carbs	Fat	
Lunch Totals							

SNACK	Time:	Amount	Calories	Protein	Carbs	Fat	
Snack Totals							

DINNER	Time:	Amount	Calories	Protein	Carbs	Fat	
Dinner Totals							

SNACK	Time:	Amount	Calories	Protein	Carbs	Fat	
Snack Totals							
DAY'S TOTALS							

Water Intake (8-oz servings)

Fruit/Vegetable Servings

Physical Activity		Duration	Calories Burned
Total Calories Burned			

Rate Your Day

① ② ③ ④ ⑤
⑥ ⑦ ⑧ ⑨ ⑩

Well Done

Keep Trying

DATE: / /

○ Mon ○ Tue ● Wed
○ Thu ● Fri ○ Sat ○ Sun

BREAKFAST Time:	Amount	Calories	Protein	Carbs	Fat	
Breakfast Totals						

SNACK Time:	Amount	Calories	Protein	Carbs	Fat	
Snack Totals						

LUNCH Time:	Amount	Calories	Protein	Carbs	Fat	
Lunch Totals						

SNACK Time:	Amount	Calories	Protein	Carbs	Fat	
Snack Totals						

DINNER	Time:	Amount	Calories	Protein	Carbs	Fat	
Dinner Totals							

SNACK	Time:	Amount	Calories	Protein	Carbs	Fat	
Snack Totals							
DAY'S TOTALS							

Water Intake (8-oz servings)

Fruit/Vegetable Servings

Physical Activity	Duration	Calories Burned
Total Calories Burned		

Rate Your Day

1 2 3 4 5
6 7 8 9 10

Well Done

Keep Trying

DATE: / /

Mon Tue **Wed**
Thu Fri Sat Sun

BREAKFAST Time:	Amount	Calories	Protein	Carbs	Fat	
Breakfast Totals						

SNACK Time:	Amount	Calories	Protein	Carbs	Fat	
Snack Totals						

LUNCH Time:	Amount	Calories	Protein	Carbs	Fat	
Lunch Totals						

SNACK Time:	Amount	Calories	Protein	Carbs	Fat	
Snack Totals						

DINNER	Time:	Amount	Calories	Protein	Carbs	Fat	
Dinner Totals							

SNACK	Time:	Amount	Calories	Protein	Carbs	Fat	
Snack Totals							
DAY'S TOTALS							

Water Intake (8-oz servings)

Fruit/Vegetable Servings

Physical Activity	Duration	Calories Burned
Total Calories Burned		

Rate Your Day

1 2 3 4 5
6 7 8 9 10

Well Done

Keep Trying

DATE: / /

○ Mon ○ Tue ● Wed
○ Thu ● Fri ○ Sat ○ Sun

BREAKFAST	Time:	Amount	Calories	Protein	Carbs	Fat	
Breakfast Totals							

SNACK	Time:	Amount	Calories	Protein	Carbs	Fat	
Snack Totals							

LUNCH	Time:	Amount	Calories	Protein	Carbs	Fat	
Lunch Totals							

SNACK	Time:	Amount	Calories	Protein	Carbs	Fat	
Snack Totals							

DINNER	Time:	Amount	Calories	Protein	Carbs	Fat	
Dinner Totals							

SNACK	Time:	Amount	Calories	Protein	Carbs	Fat	
Snack Totals							
DAY'S TOTALS							

Water Intake (8-oz servings)

Fruit/Vegetable Servings

Physical Activity	Duration	Calories Burned
Total Calories Burned		

Rate Your Day

1 2 3 4 5
6 7 8 9 10

Well Done

Keep Trying

DATE: / /

Mon Tue **Wed**
Thu Fri Sat Sun

BREAKFAST	Time:	Amount	Calories	Protein	Carbs	Fat	
Breakfast Totals							

SNACK	Time:	Amount	Calories	Protein	Carbs	Fat	
Snack Totals							

LUNCH	Time:	Amount	Calories	Protein	Carbs	Fat	
Lunch Totals							

SNACK	Time:	Amount	Calories	Protein	Carbs	Fat	
Snack Totals							

DINNER	Time:	Amount	Calories	Protein	Carbs	Fat	
Dinner Totals							

SNACK	Time:	Amount	Calories	Protein	Carbs	Fat	
Snack Totals							
DAY'S TOTALS							

Water Intake (8-oz servings)

Fruit/Vegetable Servings

Physical Activity	Duration	Calories Burned
Total Calories Burned		

Rate Your Day

1 2 3 4 5
6 7 8 9 10

Well Done

Keep Trying

DATE: / /

Mon ● Tue ● Wed
Thu ● Fri ● Sat ● Sun

BREAKFAST Time:	Amount	Calories	Protein	Carbs	Fat	
Breakfast Totals						

SNACK Time:	Amount	Calories	Protein	Carbs	Fat	
Snack Totals						

LUNCH Time:	Amount	Calories	Protein	Carbs	Fat	
Lunch Totals						

SNACK Time:	Amount	Calories	Protein	Carbs	Fat	
Snack Totals						

DINNER	Time:	Amount	Calories	Protein	Carbs	Fat	
Dinner Totals							

SNACK	Time:	Amount	Calories	Protein	Carbs	Fat	
Snack Totals							
DAY'S TOTALS							

Water Intake (8-oz servings)

Fruit/Vegetable Servings

Physical Activity	Duration	Calories Burned
Total Calories Burned		

Rate Your Day

1 2 3 4 5
6 7 8 9 10

Well Done	Keep Trying

DATE: / /

Mon Tue **Wed**

Thu Fri Sat Sun

BREAKFAST Time:	Amount	Calories	Protein	Carbs	Fat	
Breakfast Totals						

SNACK Time:	Amount	Calories	Protein	Carbs	Fat	
Snack Totals						

LUNCH Time:	Amount	Calories	Protein	Carbs	Fat	
Lunch Totals						

SNACK Time:	Amount	Calories	Protein	Carbs	Fat	
Snack Totals						

DINNER	Time:	Amount	Calories	Protein	Carbs	Fat	
Dinner Totals							

SNACK	Time:	Amount	Calories	Protein	Carbs	Fat	
Snack Totals							
DAY'S TOTALS							

Water Intake (8-oz servings)

Fruit/Vegetable Servings

Physical Activity	Duration	Calories Burned
Total Calories Burned		

Rate Your Day

① ② ③ ④ ⑤
⑥ ⑦ ⑧ ⑨ ⑩

Well Done

Keep Trying

DATE: / /

Mon Tue Wed
Thu Fri Sat Sun

BREAKFAST	Time:	Amount	Calories	Protein	Carbs	Fat	
Breakfast Totals							

SNACK	Time:	Amount	Calories	Protein	Carbs	Fat	
Snack Totals							

LUNCH	Time:	Amount	Calories	Protein	Carbs	Fat	
Lunch Totals							

SNACK	Time:	Amount	Calories	Protein	Carbs	Fat	
Snack Totals							

DINNER	Time:	Amount	Calories	Protein	Carbs	Fat	
Dinner Totals							

SNACK	Time:	Amount	Calories	Protein	Carbs	Fat	
Snack Totals							
DAY'S TOTALS							

Water Intake (8-oz servings)

Fruit/Vegetable Servings

Physical Activity	Duration	Calories Burned
Total Calories Burned		

Rate Your Day

1 2 3 4 5
6 7 8 9 10

Well Done

Keep Trying

DATE: / /

○ Mon ○ Tue ● Wed
○ Thu ● Fri ○ Sat ○ Sun

BREAKFAST	Time:	Amount	Calories	Protein	Carbs	Fat	
Breakfast Totals							

SNACK	Time:	Amount	Calories	Protein	Carbs	Fat	
Snack Totals							

LUNCH	Time:	Amount	Calories	Protein	Carbs	Fat	
Lunch Totals							

SNACK	Time:	Amount	Calories	Protein	Carbs	Fat	
Snack Totals							

DINNER	Time:	Amount	Calories	Protein	Carbs	Fat	
Dinner Totals							

SNACK	Time:	Amount	Calories	Protein	Carbs	Fat	
Snack Totals							
DAY'S TOTALS							

Water Intake (8-oz servings)

Fruit/Vegetable Servings

Physical Activity	Duration	Calories Burned
Total Calories Burned		

Rate Your Day

① ② ③ ④ ⑤
⑥ ⑦ ⑧ ⑨ ⑩

Well Done

Keep Trying

DATE: / /

Mon Tue Wed
Thu Fri Sat Sun

BREAKFAST Time:	Amount	Calories	Protein	Carbs	Fat	
Breakfast Totals						

SNACK Time:	Amount	Calories	Protein	Carbs	Fat	
Snack Totals						

LUNCH Time:	Amount	Calories	Protein	Carbs	Fat	
Lunch Totals						

SNACK Time:	Amount	Calories	Protein	Carbs	Fat	
Snack Totals						

DINNER	Time:	Amount	Calories	Protein	Carbs	Fat	
Dinner Totals							

SNACK	Time:	Amount	Calories	Protein	Carbs	Fat	
Snack Totals							
DAY'S TOTALS							

Water Intake (8-oz servings)

Fruit/Vegetable Servings

Physical Activity	Duration	Calories Burned
Total Calories Burned		

Rate Your Day

1 2 3 4 5
6 7 8 9 10

Well Done

Keep Trying

DATE: / /

○ Mon ○ Tue ● Wed
○ Thu ● Fri ○ Sat ○ Sun

BREAKFAST	Time:	Amount	Calories	Protein	Carbs	Fat	
Breakfast Totals							

SNACK	Time:	Amount	Calories	Protein	Carbs	Fat	
Snack Totals							

LUNCH	Time:	Amount	Calories	Protein	Carbs	Fat	
Lunch Totals							

SNACK	Time:	Amount	Calories	Protein	Carbs	Fat	
Snack Totals							

DINNER	Time:	Amount	Calories	Protein	Carbs	Fat	
Dinner Totals							

SNACK	Time:	Amount	Calories	Protein	Carbs	Fat	
Snack Totals							
DAY'S TOTALS							

Water Intake (8-oz servings)

Fruit/Vegetable Servings

Physical Activity	Duration	Calories Burned
Total Calories Burned		

Rate Your Day

1 2 3 4 5
6 7 8 9 10

Well Done

Keep Trying

DATE: / /

○ Mon ○ Tue ● Wed
○ Thu ● Fri ○ Sat ○ Sun

BREAKFAST	Time:	Amount	Calories	Protein	Carbs	Fat	
Breakfast Totals							

SNACK	Time:	Amount	Calories	Protein	Carbs	Fat	
Snack Totals							

LUNCH	Time:	Amount	Calories	Protein	Carbs	Fat	
Lunch Totals							

SNACK	Time:	Amount	Calories	Protein	Carbs	Fat	
Snack Totals							

DINNER	Time:	Amount	Calories	Protein	Carbs	Fat	
Dinner Totals							

SNACK	Time:	Amount	Calories	Protein	Carbs	Fat	
Snack Totals							
DAY'S TOTALS							

Water Intake (8-oz servings)

Fruit/Vegetable Servings

Physical Activity	Duration	Calories Burned
Total Calories Burned		

Rate Your Day

1 2 3 4 5
6 7 8 9 10

Well Done

Keep Trying

DATE: / /

BREAKFAST	Time:	Amount	Calories	Protein	Carbs	Fat	
Breakfast Totals							

SNACK	Time:	Amount	Calories	Protein	Carbs	Fat	
Snack Totals							

LUNCH	Time:	Amount	Calories	Protein	Carbs	Fat	
Lunch Totals							

SNACK	Time:	Amount	Calories	Protein	Carbs	Fat	
Snack Totals							

DINNER	Time:	Amount	Calories	Protein	Carbs	Fat	
Dinner Totals							

SNACK	Time:	Amount	Calories	Protein	Carbs	Fat	
Snack Totals							
DAY'S TOTALS							

Water Intake (8-oz servings)

Fruit/Vegetable Servings

Physical Activity	Duration	Calories Burned
Total Calories Burned		

Rate Your Day

1 2 3 4 5
6 7 8 9 10

Well Done

Keep Trying

DATE: / /

Mon · Tue · Wed
Thu · Fri · Sat · Sun

BREAKFAST	Time:	Amount	Calories	Protein	Carbs	Fat	
Breakfast Totals							

SNACK	Time:	Amount	Calories	Protein	Carbs	Fat	
Snack Totals							

LUNCH	Time:	Amount	Calories	Protein	Carbs	Fat	
Lunch Totals							

SNACK	Time:	Amount	Calories	Protein	Carbs	Fat	
Snack Totals							

DINNER	Time:	Amount	Calories	Protein	Carbs	Fat	
Dinner Totals							

SNACK	Time:	Amount	Calories	Protein	Carbs	Fat	
Snack Totals							
DAY'S TOTALS							

Water Intake (8-oz servings)

Fruit/Vegetable Servings

Physical Activity	Duration	Calories Burned
Total Calories Burned		

Rate Your Day

1 2 3 4 5
6 7 8 9 10

Well Done

Keep Trying

DATE: / /

Mon ● Tue ● **Wed**

Thu ● Fri ● Sat ● Sun

BREAKFAST	Time:	Amount	Calories	Protein	Carbs	Fat	
Breakfast Totals							

SNACK	Time:	Amount	Calories	Protein	Carbs	Fat	
Snack Totals							

LUNCH	Time:	Amount	Calories	Protein	Carbs	Fat	
Lunch Totals							

SNACK	Time:	Amount	Calories	Protein	Carbs	Fat	
Snack Totals							

DINNER	Time:	Amount	Calories	Protein	Carbs	Fat	
Dinner Totals							

SNACK	Time:	Amount	Calories	Protein	Carbs	Fat	
Snack Totals							
DAY'S TOTALS							

Water Intake (8-oz servings)

Fruit/Vegetable Servings

Physical Activity	Duration	Calories Burned
Total Calories Burned		

Rate Your Day

1 2 3 4 5
6 7 8 9 10

Well Done	Keep Trying

DATE: / /

Mon ● Tue ● **Wed**
Thu ● Fri ● Sat ● Sun

BREAKFAST	Time:	Amount	Calories	Protein	Carbs	Fat	
Breakfast Totals							

SNACK	Time:	Amount	Calories	Protein	Carbs	Fat	
Snack Totals							

LUNCH	Time:	Amount	Calories	Protein	Carbs	Fat	
Lunch Totals							

SNACK	Time:	Amount	Calories	Protein	Carbs	Fat	
Snack Totals							

DINNER	Time:	Amount	Calories	Protein	Carbs	Fat	
Dinner Totals							

SNACK	Time:	Amount	Calories	Protein	Carbs	Fat	
Snack Totals							
DAY'S TOTALS							

Water Intake (8-oz servings)

Fruit/Vegetable Servings

Physical Activity	Duration	Calories Burned
Total Calories Burned		

Rate Your Day

① ② ③ ④ ⑤
⑥ ⑦ ⑧ ⑨ ⑩

Well Done

Keep Trying

DATE: / /

Mon Tue **Wed**
Thu Fri Sat Sun

BREAKFAST	Time:	Amount	Calories	Protein	Carbs	Fat	
Breakfast Totals							

SNACK	Time:	Amount	Calories	Protein	Carbs	Fat	
Snack Totals							

LUNCH	Time:	Amount	Calories	Protein	Carbs	Fat	
Lunch Totals							

SNACK	Time:	Amount	Calories	Protein	Carbs	Fat	
Snack Totals							

DINNER	Time:	Amount	Calories	Protein	Carbs	Fat	
Dinner Totals							

SNACK	Time:	Amount	Calories	Protein	Carbs	Fat	
Snack Totals							
DAY'S TOTALS							

Water Intake (8-oz servings)

Fruit/Vegetable Servings

Physical Activity	Duration	Calories Burned
Total Calories Burned		

Rate Your Day

1 2 3 4 5
6 7 8 9 10

Well Done

Keep Trying

DATE: / /

○ Mon ○ Tue ● Wed
○ Thu ● Fri ○ Sat ○ Sun

BREAKFAST Time:	Amount	Calories	Protein	Carbs	Fat	
Breakfast Totals						

SNACK Time:	Amount	Calories	Protein	Carbs	Fat	
Snack Totals						

LUNCH Time:	Amount	Calories	Protein	Carbs	Fat	
Lunch Totals						

SNACK Time:	Amount	Calories	Protein	Carbs	Fat	
Snack Totals						

MY FOOD JOURNAL

DINNER	Time:	Amount	Calories	Protein	Carbs	Fat	
Dinner Totals							

SNACK	Time:	Amount	Calories	Protein	Carbs	Fat	
Snack Totals							
DAY'S TOTALS							

Water Intake (8-oz servings)

Fruit/Vegetable Servings

Physical Activity	Duration	Calories Burned
Total Calories Burned		

Rate Your Day

① ② ③ ④ ⑤
⑥ ⑦ ⑧ ⑨ ⑩

Well Done

Keep Trying

DATE: / /

○ Mon ○ Tue ● Wed
○ Thu ● Fri ○ Sat ○ Sun

BREAKFAST	Time:	Amount	Calories	Protein	Carbs	Fat	
Breakfast Totals							

SNACK	Time:	Amount	Calories	Protein	Carbs	Fat	
Snack Totals							

LUNCH	Time:	Amount	Calories	Protein	Carbs	Fat	
Lunch Totals							

SNACK	Time:	Amount	Calories	Protein	Carbs	Fat	
Snack Totals							

DINNER	Time:	Amount	Calories	Protein	Carbs	Fat	
Dinner Totals							

SNACK	Time:	Amount	Calories	Protein	Carbs	Fat	
Snack Totals							
DAY'S TOTALS							

Water Intake (8-oz servings)

Fruit/Vegetable Servings

Physical Activity	Duration	Calories Burned
Total Calories Burned		

Rate Your Day

① ② ③ ④ ⑤
⑥ ⑦ ⑧ ⑨ ⑩

Well Done

Keep Trying

DATE: / /

Mon Tue **Wed**
Thu Fri Sat Sun

BREAKFAST	Time:	Amount	Calories	Protein	Carbs	Fat	
Breakfast Totals							

SNACK	Time:	Amount	Calories	Protein	Carbs	Fat	
Snack Totals							

LUNCH	Time:	Amount	Calories	Protein	Carbs	Fat	
Lunch Totals							

SNACK	Time:	Amount	Calories	Protein	Carbs	Fat	
Snack Totals							

DINNER	Time:	Amount	Calories	Protein	Carbs	Fat	
Dinner Totals							

SNACK	Time:	Amount	Calories	Protein	Carbs	Fat	
Snack Totals							
DAY'S TOTALS							

Water Intake (8-oz servings)

Fruit/Vegetable Servings

Physical Activity	Duration	Calories Burned
Total Calories Burned		

Rate Your Day

1 2 3 4 5
6 7 8 9 10

Well Done

Keep Trying

DATE: / /

Mon ○ Tue ● Wed
○ Thu ● Fri ○ Sat ○ Sun

BREAKFAST Time:	Amount	Calories	Protein	Carbs	Fat	
Breakfast Totals						

SNACK Time:	Amount	Calories	Protein	Carbs	Fat	
Snack Totals						

LUNCH Time:	Amount	Calories	Protein	Carbs	Fat	
Lunch Totals						

SNACK Time:	Amount	Calories	Protein	Carbs	Fat	
Snack Totals						

DINNER	Time:	Amount	Calories	Protein	Carbs	Fat	
Dinner Totals							

SNACK	Time:	Amount	Calories	Protein	Carbs	Fat	
Snack Totals							
DAY'S TOTALS							

Water Intake (8-oz servings)

Fruit/Vegetable Servings

Physical Activity	Duration	Calories Burned
Total Calories Burned		

Rate Your Day

1 2 3 4 5
6 7 8 9 10

Well Done

Keep Trying

DATE: / /

○ Mon ○ Tue ● Wed
○ Thu ● Fri ○ Sat ○ Sun

BREAKFAST	Time:	Amount	Calories	Protein	Carbs	Fat	
Breakfast Totals							

SNACK	Time:	Amount	Calories	Protein	Carbs	Fat	
Snack Totals							

LUNCH	Time:	Amount	Calories	Protein	Carbs	Fat	
Lunch Totals							

SNACK	Time:	Amount	Calories	Protein	Carbs	Fat	
Snack Totals							

DINNER	Time:	Amount	Calories	Protein	Carbs	Fat	
Dinner Totals							

SNACK	Time:	Amount	Calories	Protein	Carbs	Fat	
Snack Totals							
DAY'S TOTALS							

Water Intake (8-oz servings)

Fruit/Vegetable Servings

Physical Activity	Duration	Calories Burned
Total Calories Burned		

Rate Your Day

1 2 3 4 5
6 7 8 9 10

Well Done

Keep Trying

DATE: / /

○ Mon ○ Tue ● Wed
○ Thu ○ Fri ○ Sat ○ Sun

BREAKFAST Time:	Amount	Calories	Protein	Carbs	Fat	
Breakfast Totals						

SNACK Time:	Amount	Calories	Protein	Carbs	Fat	
Snack Totals						

LUNCH Time:	Amount	Calories	Protein	Carbs	Fat	
Lunch Totals						

SNACK Time:	Amount	Calories	Protein	Carbs	Fat	
Snack Totals						

DINNER	Time:	Amount	Calories	Protein	Carbs	Fat	
Dinner Totals							

SNACK	Time:	Amount	Calories	Protein	Carbs	Fat	
Snack Totals							
DAY'S TOTALS							

Water Intake (8-oz servings)

Fruit/Vegetable Servings

Physical Activity	Duration	Calories Burned
Total Calories Burned		

Rate Your Day

1 2 3 4 5
6 7 8 9 10

Well Done

Keep Trying

DATE: / /

○ Mon ○ Tue ● Wed
○ Thu ● Fri ○ Sat ○ Sun

BREAKFAST	Time:	Amount	Calories	Protein	Carbs	Fat	
Breakfast Totals							

SNACK	Time:	Amount	Calories	Protein	Carbs	Fat	
Snack Totals							

LUNCH	Time:	Amount	Calories	Protein	Carbs	Fat	
Lunch Totals							

SNACK	Time:	Amount	Calories	Protein	Carbs	Fat	
Snack Totals							

DINNER	Time:	Amount	Calories	Protein	Carbs	Fat	
Dinner Totals							

SNACK	Time:	Amount	Calories	Protein	Carbs	Fat	
Snack Totals							
DAY'S TOTALS							

Water Intake (8-oz servings)

Fruit/Vegetable Servings

Physical Activity	Duration	Calories Burned
Total Calories Burned		

Rate Your Day

1 2 3 4 5
6 7 8 9 10

Well Done

Keep Trying

DATE: / /

○ Mon ○ Tue ● Wed
○ Thu ● Fri ○ Sat ○ Sun

BREAKFAST Time:	Amount	Calories	Protein	Carbs	Fat	
Breakfast Totals						

SNACK Time:	Amount	Calories	Protein	Carbs	Fat	
Snack Totals						

LUNCH Time:	Amount	Calories	Protein	Carbs	Fat	
Lunch Totals						

SNACK Time:	Amount	Calories	Protein	Carbs	Fat	
Snack Totals						

MY FOOD JOURNAL

DINNER	Time:	Amount	Calories	Protein	Carbs	Fat	
Dinner Totals							

SNACK	Time:	Amount	Calories	Protein	Carbs	Fat	
Snack Totals							
DAY'S TOTALS							

Water Intake (8-oz servings)

Fruit/Vegetable Servings

Physical Activity		Duration		Calories Burned
Total Calories Burned				

Rate Your Day

1 2 3 4 5
6 7 8 9 10

Well Done

Keep Trying

DATE: / /

Mon ● Tue ● Wed
Thu ● Fri ● Sat ● Sun

BREAKFAST	Time:	Amount	Calories	Protein	Carbs	Fat	
Breakfast Totals							

SNACK	Time:	Amount	Calories	Protein	Carbs	Fat	
Snack Totals							

LUNCH	Time:	Amount	Calories	Protein	Carbs	Fat	
Lunch Totals							

SNACK	Time:	Amount	Calories	Protein	Carbs	Fat	
Snack Totals							

DINNER	Time:	Amount	Calories	Protein	Carbs	Fat	
Dinner Totals							

SNACK	Time:	Amount	Calories	Protein	Carbs	Fat	
Snack Totals							
DAY'S TOTALS							

Water Intake (8-oz servings)

Fruit/Vegetable Servings

Physical Activity	Duration	Calories Burned
Total Calories Burned		

Rate Your Day

1 2 3 4 5
6 7 8 9 10

Well Done

Keep Trying

DATE: / /

Mon ● Tue ● Wed ●
Thu ● Fri ● Sat ● Sun ●

BREAKFAST	Time:	Amount	Calories	Protein	Carbs	Fat	
Breakfast Totals							

SNACK	Time:	Amount	Calories	Protein	Carbs	Fat	
Snack Totals							

LUNCH	Time:	Amount	Calories	Protein	Carbs	Fat	
Lunch Totals							

SNACK	Time:	Amount	Calories	Protein	Carbs	Fat	
Snack Totals							

DINNER	Time:	Amount	Calories	Protein	Carbs	Fat	
Dinner Totals							

SNACK	Time:	Amount	Calories	Protein	Carbs	Fat	
Snack Totals							
DAY'S TOTALS							

Water Intake (8-oz servings)

Fruit/Vegetable Servings

Physical Activity	Duration	Calories Burned
Total Calories Burned		

Rate Your Day

1 2 3 4 5
6 7 8 9 10

Well Done

Keep Trying

DATE: / /

○ Mon ○ Tue ● Wed
○ Thu ○ Fri ○ Sat ○ Sun

BREAKFAST Time:	Amount	Calories	Protein	Carbs	Fat	
Breakfast Totals						

SNACK Time:	Amount	Calories	Protein	Carbs	Fat	
Snack Totals						

LUNCH Time:	Amount	Calories	Protein	Carbs	Fat	
Lunch Totals						

SNACK Time:	Amount	Calories	Protein	Carbs	Fat	
Snack Totals						

DINNER	Time:	Amount	Calories	Protein	Carbs	Fat	
Dinner Totals							

SNACK	Time:	Amount	Calories	Protein	Carbs	Fat	
Snack Totals							
DAY'S TOTALS							

Water Intake (8-oz servings)

Fruit/Vegetable Servings

Physical Activity	Duration	Calories Burned
Total Calories Burned		

Rate Your Day

1 2 3 4 5
6 7 8 9 10

Well Done

Keep Trying

DATE: / /

○ Mon ○ Tue ● Wed
○ Thu ○ Fri ○ Sat ○ Sun

BREAKFAST	Time:	Amount	Calories	Protein	Carbs	Fat	
Breakfast Totals							

SNACK	Time:	Amount	Calories	Protein	Carbs	Fat	
Snack Totals							

LUNCH	Time:	Amount	Calories	Protein	Carbs	Fat	
Lunch Totals							

SNACK	Time:	Amount	Calories	Protein	Carbs	Fat	
Snack Totals							

DINNER	Time:	Amount	Calories	Protein	Carbs	Fat	
Dinner Totals							

SNACK	Time:	Amount	Calories	Protein	Carbs	Fat	
Snack Totals							
DAY'S TOTALS							

Water Intake (8-oz servings)

Fruit/Vegetable Servings

Physical Activity	Duration	Calories Burned
Total Calories Burned		

Rate Your Day

1 2 3 4 5
6 7 8 9 10

Well Done

Keep Trying

DATE: / /

○ Mon ○ Tue ● Wed
○ Thu ● Fri ○ Sat ○ Sun

BREAKFAST	Time:	Amount	Calories	Protein	Carbs	Fat	
Breakfast Totals							

SNACK	Time:	Amount	Calories	Protein	Carbs	Fat	
Snack Totals							

LUNCH	Time:	Amount	Calories	Protein	Carbs	Fat	
Lunch Totals							

SNACK	Time:	Amount	Calories	Protein	Carbs	Fat	
Snack Totals							

DINNER	Time:	Amount	Calories	Protein	Carbs	Fat	
Dinner Totals							

SNACK	Time:	Amount	Calories	Protein	Carbs	Fat	
Snack Totals							
DAY'S TOTALS							

Water Intake (8-oz servings)

Fruit/Vegetable Servings

Physical Activity	Duration	Calories Burned
Total Calories Burned		

Rate Your Day

1 2 3 4 5
6 7 8 9 10

Well Done

Keep Trying

DATE: / /

Mon Tue **Wed**
Thu Fri Sat Sun

BREAKFAST	Time:	Amount	Calories	Protein	Carbs	Fat	
Breakfast Totals							

SNACK	Time:	Amount	Calories	Protein	Carbs	Fat	
Snack Totals							

LUNCH	Time:	Amount	Calories	Protein	Carbs	Fat	
Lunch Totals							

SNACK	Time:	Amount	Calories	Protein	Carbs	Fat	
Snack Totals							

DINNER	Time:	Amount	Calories	Protein	Carbs	Fat	
Dinner Totals							

SNACK	Time:	Amount	Calories	Protein	Carbs	Fat	
Snack Totals							
DAY'S TOTALS							

Water Intake (8-oz servings)

Fruit/Vegetable Servings

Physical Activity	Duration	Calories Burned
Total Calories Burned		

Rate Your Day

1 2 3 4 5
6 7 8 9 10

Well Done	Keep Trying

DATE: / /

Mon ● Tue ● Wed
Thu ● Fri ● Sat ● Sun

BREAKFAST Time:	Amount	Calories	Protein	Carbs	Fat	
Breakfast Totals						

SNACK Time:	Amount	Calories	Protein	Carbs	Fat	
Snack Totals						

LUNCH Time:	Amount	Calories	Protein	Carbs	Fat	
Lunch Totals						

SNACK Time:	Amount	Calories	Protein	Carbs	Fat	
Snack Totals						

DINNER	Time:	Amount	Calories	Protein	Carbs	Fat	
Dinner Totals							

SNACK	Time:	Amount	Calories	Protein	Carbs	Fat	
Snack Totals							
DAY'S TOTALS							

Water Intake (8-oz servings)

Fruit/Vegetable Servings

Physical Activity	Duration	Calories Burned
Total Calories Burned		

Rate Your Day

1 2 3 4 5
6 7 8 9 10

Well Done

Keep Trying

DATE: / /

○ Mon ○ Tue ● Wed
○ Thu ● Fri ○ Sat ○ Sun

BREAKFAST	Time:	Amount	Calories	Protein	Carbs	Fat	
Breakfast Totals							

SNACK	Time:	Amount	Calories	Protein	Carbs	Fat	
Snack Totals							

LUNCH	Time:	Amount	Calories	Protein	Carbs	Fat	
Lunch Totals							

SNACK	Time:	Amount	Calories	Protein	Carbs	Fat	
Snack Totals							

DINNER	Time:	Amount	Calories	Protein	Carbs	Fat	
Dinner Totals							

SNACK	Time:	Amount	Calories	Protein	Carbs	Fat	
Snack Totals							
DAY'S TOTALS							

Water Intake (8-oz servings)

Fruit/Vegetable Servings

Physical Activity	Duration	Calories Burned
Total Calories Burned		

Rate Your Day

1 2 3 4 5
6 7 8 9 10

Well Done

Keep Trying

DATE: / /

Mon Tue **Wed**
Thu Fri Sat Sun

BREAKFAST	Time:	Amount	Calories	Protein	Carbs	Fat	
Breakfast Totals							

SNACK	Time:	Amount	Calories	Protein	Carbs	Fat	
Snack Totals							

LUNCH	Time:	Amount	Calories	Protein	Carbs	Fat	
Lunch Totals							

SNACK	Time:	Amount	Calories	Protein	Carbs	Fat	
Snack Totals							

DINNER	Time:	Amount	Calories	Protein	Carbs	Fat	
Dinner Totals							

SNACK	Time:	Amount	Calories	Protein	Carbs	Fat	
Snack Totals							
DAY'S TOTALS							

Water Intake (8-oz servings)

Fruit/Vegetable Servings

Physical Activity	Duration	Calories Burned
Total Calories Burned		

Rate Your Day

1 2 3 4 5
6 7 8 9 10

Well Done

Keep Trying

DATE: / /

Mon ● Tue ● **Wed**
Thu ● Fri ● Sat ● Sun

BREAKFAST	Time:	Amount	Calories	Protein	Carbs	Fat	
Breakfast Totals							

SNACK	Time:	Amount	Calories	Protein	Carbs	Fat	
Snack Totals							

LUNCH	Time:	Amount	Calories	Protein	Carbs	Fat	
Lunch Totals							

SNACK	Time:	Amount	Calories	Protein	Carbs	Fat	
Snack Totals							

DINNER	Time:	Amount	Calories	Protein	Carbs	Fat	
Dinner Totals							

SNACK	Time:	Amount	Calories	Protein	Carbs	Fat	
Snack Totals							
DAY'S TOTALS							

Water Intake (8-oz servings)

Fruit/Vegetable Servings

Physical Activity	Duration	Calories Burned
Total Calories Burned		

Rate Your Day

1 2 3 4 5
6 7 8 9 10

Well Done

Keep Trying

DATE: / /

◯ Mon ◯ Tue ● Wed
◯ Thu ◯ Fri ◯ Sat ◯ Sun

BREAKFAST	Time:	Amount	Calories	Protein	Carbs	Fat	
Breakfast Totals							

SNACK	Time:	Amount	Calories	Protein	Carbs	Fat	
Snack Totals							

LUNCH	Time:	Amount	Calories	Protein	Carbs	Fat	
Lunch Totals							

SNACK	Time:	Amount	Calories	Protein	Carbs	Fat	
Snack Totals							

DINNER	Time:	Amount	Calories	Protein	Carbs	Fat	
Dinner Totals							

SNACK	Time:	Amount	Calories	Protein	Carbs	Fat	
Snack Totals							
DAY'S TOTALS							

Water Intake (8-oz servings)

Fruit/Vegetable Servings

Physical Activity	Duration	Calories Burned
Total Calories Burned		

Rate Your Day

1 2 3 4 5
6 7 8 9 10

Well Done

Keep Trying

DATE: / /

○ Mon ○ Tue ● Wed
○ Thu ○ Fri ○ Sat ○ Sun

BREAKFAST	Time:	Amount	Calories	Protein	Carbs	Fat	
Breakfast Totals							

SNACK	Time:	Amount	Calories	Protein	Carbs	Fat	
Snack Totals							

LUNCH	Time:	Amount	Calories	Protein	Carbs	Fat	
Lunch Totals							

SNACK	Time:	Amount	Calories	Protein	Carbs	Fat	
Snack Totals							

DINNER	Time:	Amount	Calories	Protein	Carbs	Fat	
Dinner Totals							

SNACK	Time:	Amount	Calories	Protein	Carbs	Fat	
Snack Totals							
DAY'S TOTALS							

Water Intake (8-oz servings)

Fruit/Vegetable Servings

Physical Activity	Duration	Calories Burned
Total Calories Burned		

Rate Your Day

1 2 3 4 5
6 7 8 9 10

Well Done

Keep Trying

DATE: / /

○ Mon ○ Tue ● Wed
○ Thu ● Fri ○ Sat ○ Sun

BREAKFAST	Time:	Amount	Calories	Protein	Carbs	Fat	
Breakfast Totals							

SNACK	Time:	Amount	Calories	Protein	Carbs	Fat	
Snack Totals							

LUNCH	Time:	Amount	Calories	Protein	Carbs	Fat	
Lunch Totals							

SNACK	Time:	Amount	Calories	Protein	Carbs	Fat	
Snack Totals							

DINNER	Time:	Amount	Calories	Protein	Carbs	Fat	
Dinner Totals							

SNACK	Time:	Amount	Calories	Protein	Carbs	Fat	
Snack Totals							
DAY'S TOTALS							

Water Intake (8-oz servings)

Fruit/Vegetable Servings

Physical Activity	Duration	Calories Burned
Total Calories Burned		

Rate Your Day

1 2 3 4 5
6 7 8 9 10

Well Done	Keep Trying

DATE: / /

○ Mon ○ Tue ● Wed
○ Thu ● Fri ○ Sat ○ Sun

BREAKFAST	Time:	Amount	Calories	Protein	Carbs	Fat	
Breakfast Totals							

SNACK	Time:	Amount	Calories	Protein	Carbs	Fat	
Snack Totals							

LUNCH	Time:	Amount	Calories	Protein	Carbs	Fat	
Lunch Totals							

SNACK	Time:	Amount	Calories	Protein	Carbs	Fat	
Snack Totals							

DINNER	Time:	Amount	Calories	Protein	Carbs	Fat	
Dinner Totals							

SNACK	Time:	Amount	Calories	Protein	Carbs	Fat	
Snack Totals							
DAY'S TOTALS							

Water Intake (8-oz servings)

Fruit/Vegetable Servings

Physical Activity	Duration	Calories Burned
Total Calories Burned		

Rate Your Day

① ② ③ ④ ⑤
⑥ ⑦ ⑧ ⑨ ⑩

Well Done

Keep Trying

DATE: / /

Mon ● Tue ● Wed ●
Thu ● Fri ● Sat ● Sun ●

BREAKFAST	Time:	Amount	Calories	Protein	Carbs	Fat	
Breakfast Totals							

SNACK	Time:	Amount	Calories	Protein	Carbs	Fat	
Snack Totals							

LUNCH	Time:	Amount	Calories	Protein	Carbs	Fat	
Lunch Totals							

SNACK	Time:	Amount	Calories	Protein	Carbs	Fat	
Snack Totals							

DINNER	Time:	Amount	Calories	Protein	Carbs	Fat	
Dinner Totals							

SNACK	Time:	Amount	Calories	Protein	Carbs	Fat	
Snack Totals							
DAY'S TOTALS							

Water Intake (8-oz servings)

Fruit/Vegetable Servings

Physical Activity	Duration	Calories Burned
Total Calories Burned		

Rate Your Day

1 2 3 4 5
6 7 8 9 10

Well Done	Keep Trying

DATE: / /

Mon ● Tue ● Wed
Thu ● Fri ● Sat ● Sun

BREAKFAST	Time:	Amount	Calories	Protein	Carbs	Fat	
Breakfast Totals							

SNACK	Time:	Amount	Calories	Protein	Carbs	Fat	
Snack Totals							

LUNCH	Time:	Amount	Calories	Protein	Carbs	Fat	
Lunch Totals							

SNACK	Time:	Amount	Calories	Protein	Carbs	Fat	
Snack Totals							

DINNER	Time:	Amount	Calories	Protein	Carbs	Fat	
Dinner Totals							

SNACK	Time:	Amount	Calories	Protein	Carbs	Fat	
Snack Totals							
DAY'S TOTALS							

Water Intake (8-oz servings)

Fruit/Vegetable Servings

Physical Activity	Duration	Calories Burned
Total Calories Burned		

Rate Your Day

1 2 3 4 5
6 7 8 9 10

Well Done

Keep Trying

DATE: / /

○ Mon ○ Tue ● Wed
○ Thu ○ Fri ○ Sat ○ Sun

BREAKFAST	Time:	Amount	Calories	Protein	Carbs	Fat	
Breakfast Totals							

SNACK	Time:	Amount	Calories	Protein	Carbs	Fat	
Snack Totals							

LUNCH	Time:	Amount	Calories	Protein	Carbs	Fat	
Lunch Totals							

SNACK	Time:	Amount	Calories	Protein	Carbs	Fat	
Snack Totals							

DINNER	Time:	Amount	Calories	Protein	Carbs	Fat	
Dinner Totals							

SNACK	Time:	Amount	Calories	Protein	Carbs	Fat	
Snack Totals							
DAY'S TOTALS							

Water Intake (8-oz servings)

Fruit/Vegetable Servings

Physical Activity	Duration	Calories Burned
Total Calories Burned		

Rate Your Day

1 2 3 4 5
6 7 8 9 10

Well Done

Keep Trying

DATE: / /

Mon Tue **Wed**

Thu Fri Sat Sun

BREAKFAST	Time:	Amount	Calories	Protein	Carbs	Fat	
Breakfast Totals							

SNACK	Time:	Amount	Calories	Protein	Carbs	Fat	
Snack Totals							

LUNCH	Time:	Amount	Calories	Protein	Carbs	Fat	
Lunch Totals							

SNACK	Time:	Amount	Calories	Protein	Carbs	Fat	
Snack Totals							

DINNER	Time:	Amount	Calories	Protein	Carbs	Fat	
Dinner Totals							

SNACK	Time:	Amount	Calories	Protein	Carbs	Fat	
Snack Totals							
DAY'S TOTALS							

Water Intake (8-oz servings)

Fruit/Vegetable Servings

Physical Activity	Duration	Calories Burned
Total Calories Burned		

Rate Your Day

1 2 3 4 5
6 7 8 9 10

Well Done

Keep Trying

DATE: / /

● Mon ● Tue ● Wed
● Thu ● Fri ● Sat ● Sun

BREAKFAST	Time:	Amount	Calories	Protein	Carbs	Fat	
Breakfast Totals							

SNACK	Time:	Amount	Calories	Protein	Carbs	Fat	
Snack Totals							

LUNCH	Time:	Amount	Calories	Protein	Carbs	Fat	
Lunch Totals							

SNACK	Time:	Amount	Calories	Protein	Carbs	Fat	
Snack Totals							

DINNER	Time:	Amount	Calories	Protein	Carbs	Fat	
Dinner Totals							

SNACK	Time:	Amount	Calories	Protein	Carbs	Fat	
Snack Totals							
DAY'S TOTALS							

Water Intake (8-oz servings)

Fruit/Vegetable Servings

Physical Activity		Duration	Calories Burned
Total Calories Burned			

Rate Your Day

1 2 3 4 5
6 7 8 9 10

Well Done

Keep Trying

DATE: / /

Mon ● Tue ● **Wed** ●

Thu ● Fri ● Sat ● Sun ●

BREAKFAST	Time:	Amount	Calories	Protein	Carbs	Fat	
Breakfast Totals							

SNACK	Time:	Amount	Calories	Protein	Carbs	Fat	
Snack Totals							

LUNCH	Time:	Amount	Calories	Protein	Carbs	Fat	
Lunch Totals							

SNACK	Time:	Amount	Calories	Protein	Carbs	Fat	
Snack Totals							

DINNER	Time:	Amount	Calories	Protein	Carbs	Fat	
Dinner Totals							

SNACK	Time:	Amount	Calories	Protein	Carbs	Fat	
Snack Totals							
DAY'S TOTALS							

Water Intake (8-oz servings)

Fruit/Vegetable Servings

Physical Activity	Duration	Calories Burned
Total Calories Burned		

Rate Your Day

1 2 3 4 5
6 7 8 9 10

Well Done

Keep Trying

DATE: / /

Mon ● Tue ● Wed
Thu ● Fri ● Sat ● Sun

BREAKFAST	Time:	Amount	Calories	Protein	Carbs	Fat	
Breakfast Totals							

SNACK	Time:	Amount	Calories	Protein	Carbs	Fat	
Snack Totals							

LUNCH	Time:	Amount	Calories	Protein	Carbs	Fat	
Lunch Totals							

SNACK	Time:	Amount	Calories	Protein	Carbs	Fat	
Snack Totals							

DINNER	Time:	Amount	Calories	Protein	Carbs	Fat	
Dinner Totals							

SNACK	Time:	Amount	Calories	Protein	Carbs	Fat	
Snack Totals							
DAY'S TOTALS							

Water Intake (8-oz servings)

Fruit/Vegetable Servings

Physical Activity	Duration	Calories Burned
Total Calories Burned		

Rate Your Day

1 2 3 4 5
6 7 8 9 10

Well Done	Keep Trying

DATE: / /

Mon ◯ Tue ● Wed
Thu ● Fri ◯ Sat ◯ Sun

BREAKFAST	Time:	Amount	Calories	Protein	Carbs	Fat	
Breakfast Totals							

SNACK	Time:	Amount	Calories	Protein	Carbs	Fat	
Snack Totals							

LUNCH	Time:	Amount	Calories	Protein	Carbs	Fat	
Lunch Totals							

SNACK	Time:	Amount	Calories	Protein	Carbs	Fat	
Snack Totals							

DINNER	Time:	Amount	Calories	Protein	Carbs	Fat	
Dinner Totals							

SNACK	Time:	Amount	Calories	Protein	Carbs	Fat	
Snack Totals							
DAY'S TOTALS							

Water Intake (8-oz servings)

Fruit/Vegetable Servings

Physical Activity	Duration	Calories Burned
Total Calories Burned		

Rate Your Day

1 2 3 4 5
6 7 8 9 10

Well Done

Keep Trying

DATE: / /

Mon ● Tue ● Wed
Thu ● Fri ● Sat ● Sun

BREAKFAST	Time:	Amount	Calories	Protein	Carbs	Fat	
Breakfast Totals							

SNACK	Time:	Amount	Calories	Protein	Carbs	Fat	
Snack Totals							

LUNCH	Time:	Amount	Calories	Protein	Carbs	Fat	
Lunch Totals							

SNACK	Time:	Amount	Calories	Protein	Carbs	Fat	
Snack Totals							

DINNER	Time:	Amount	Calories	Protein	Carbs	Fat	
Dinner Totals							

SNACK	Time:	Amount	Calories	Protein	Carbs	Fat	
Snack Totals							
DAY'S TOTALS							

Water Intake (8-oz servings)

Fruit/Vegetable Servings

Physical Activity	Duration	Calories Burned
Total Calories Burned		

Rate Your Day

1 2 3 4 5
6 7 8 9 10

Well Done

Keep Trying

DATE: / /

○ Mon ○ Tue ● Wed
○ Thu ● Fri ○ Sat ○ Sun

BREAKFAST	Time:	Amount	Calories	Protein	Carbs	Fat	
Breakfast Totals							

SNACK	Time:	Amount	Calories	Protein	Carbs	Fat	
Snack Totals							

LUNCH	Time:	Amount	Calories	Protein	Carbs	Fat	
Lunch Totals							

SNACK	Time:	Amount	Calories	Protein	Carbs	Fat	
Snack Totals							

DINNER	Time:	Amount	Calories	Protein	Carbs	Fat	
Dinner Totals							

SNACK	Time:	Amount	Calories	Protein	Carbs	Fat	
Snack Totals							
DAY'S TOTALS							

Water Intake (8-oz servings)

Fruit/Vegetable Servings

Physical Activity	Duration	Calories Burned
Total Calories Burned		

Rate Your Day

1 2 3 4 5
6 7 8 9 10

Well Done

Keep Trying

DATE: / /

Mon Tue **Wed**
Thu Fri Sat Sun

BREAKFAST	Time:	Amount	Calories	Protein	Carbs	Fat	
Breakfast Totals							

SNACK	Time:	Amount	Calories	Protein	Carbs	Fat	
Snack Totals							

LUNCH	Time:	Amount	Calories	Protein	Carbs	Fat	
Lunch Totals							

SNACK	Time:	Amount	Calories	Protein	Carbs	Fat	
Snack Totals							

DINNER	Time:	Amount	Calories	Protein	Carbs	Fat	
Dinner Totals							

SNACK	Time:	Amount	Calories	Protein	Carbs	Fat	
Snack Totals							
DAY'S TOTALS							

Water Intake (8-oz servings)

Fruit/Vegetable Servings

Physical Activity	Duration	Calories Burned
Total Calories Burned		

Rate Your Day

1 2 3 4 5
6 7 8 9 10

Well Done

Keep Trying

DATE: / /

Mon Tue **Wed**
Thu Fri Sat Sun

BREAKFAST Time:	Amount	Calories	Protein	Carbs	Fat	
Breakfast Totals						

SNACK Time:	Amount	Calories	Protein	Carbs	Fat	
Snack Totals						

LUNCH Time:	Amount	Calories	Protein	Carbs	Fat	
Lunch Totals						

SNACK Time:	Amount	Calories	Protein	Carbs	Fat	
Snack Totals						

DINNER	Time:	Amount	Calories	Protein	Carbs	Fat	
Dinner Totals							

SNACK	Time:	Amount	Calories	Protein	Carbs	Fat	
Snack Totals							
DAY'S TOTALS							

Water Intake (8-oz servings)

Fruit/Vegetable Servings

Physical Activity	Duration	Calories Burned
Total Calories Burned		

Rate Your Day

1 2 3 4 5
6 7 8 9 10

Well Done

Keep Trying

DATE: / /

○ Mon ○ Tue ● Wed
○ Thu ● Fri ○ Sat ○ Sun

BREAKFAST Time:	Amount	Calories	Protein	Carbs	Fat	
Breakfast Totals						

SNACK Time:	Amount	Calories	Protein	Carbs	Fat	
Snack Totals						

LUNCH Time:	Amount	Calories	Protein	Carbs	Fat	
Lunch Totals						

SNACK Time:	Amount	Calories	Protein	Carbs	Fat	
Snack Totals						

DINNER	Time:	Amount	Calories	Protein	Carbs	Fat	
Dinner Totals							

SNACK	Time:	Amount	Calories	Protein	Carbs	Fat	
Snack Totals							
DAY'S TOTALS							

Water Intake (8-oz servings)

Fruit/Vegetable Servings

Physical Activity		Duration	Calories Burned
Total Calories Burned			

Rate Your Day

① ② ③ ④ ⑤
⑥ ⑦ ⑧ ⑨ ⑩

Well Done

Keep Trying

DATE: / /

○ Mon ○ Tue ● Wed
○ Thu ○ Fri ○ Sat ○ Sun

BREAKFAST	Time:	Amount	Calories	Protein	Carbs	Fat	
Breakfast Totals							

SNACK	Time:	Amount	Calories	Protein	Carbs	Fat	
Snack Totals							

LUNCH	Time:	Amount	Calories	Protein	Carbs	Fat	
Lunch Totals							

SNACK	Time:	Amount	Calories	Protein	Carbs	Fat	
Snack Totals							

DINNER	Time:	Amount	Calories	Protein	Carbs	Fat	
Dinner Totals							

SNACK	Time:	Amount	Calories	Protein	Carbs	Fat	
Snack Totals							
DAY'S TOTALS							

Water Intake (8-oz servings)

Fruit/Vegetable Servings

Physical Activity	Duration	Calories Burned
Total Calories Burned		

Rate Your Day

1 2 3 4 5
6 7 8 9 10

Well Done

Keep Trying

DATE: / /

○ Mon ○ Tue ● Wed
○ Thu ● Fri ○ Sat ○ Sun

BREAKFAST	Time:	Amount	Calories	Protein	Carbs	Fat	
Breakfast Totals							

SNACK	Time:	Amount	Calories	Protein	Carbs	Fat	
Snack Totals							

LUNCH	Time:	Amount	Calories	Protein	Carbs	Fat	
Lunch Totals							

SNACK	Time:	Amount	Calories	Protein	Carbs	Fat	
Snack Totals							

DINNER	Time:	Amount	Calories	Protein	Carbs	Fat	
Dinner Totals							

SNACK	Time:	Amount	Calories	Protein	Carbs	Fat	
Snack Totals							
DAY'S TOTALS							

Water Intake (8-oz servings)

Fruit/Vegetable Servings

Physical Activity	Duration	Calories Burned
Total Calories Burned		

Rate Your Day

1 2 3 4 5
6 7 8 9 10

Well Done

Keep Trying

DATE: / /

○ Mon ○ Tue ● Wed
○ Thu ● Fri ○ Sat ○ Sun

BREAKFAST	Time:	Amount	Calories	Protein	Carbs	Fat	
Breakfast Totals							

SNACK	Time:	Amount	Calories	Protein	Carbs	Fat	
Snack Totals							

LUNCH	Time:	Amount	Calories	Protein	Carbs	Fat	
Lunch Totals							

SNACK	Time:	Amount	Calories	Protein	Carbs	Fat	
Snack Totals							

DINNER	Time:	Amount	Calories	Protein	Carbs	Fat	
Dinner Totals							

SNACK	Time:	Amount	Calories	Protein	Carbs	Fat	
Snack Totals							
DAY'S TOTALS							

Water Intake (8-oz servings)

Fruit/Vegetable Servings

Physical Activity	Duration	Calories Burned
Total Calories Burned		

Rate Your Day

1 2 3 4 5
6 7 8 9 10

Well Done

Keep Trying

DATE: / /

○ Mon ○ Tue ● Wed
○ Thu ● Fri ○ Sat ○ Sun

BREAKFAST	Time:	Amount	Calories	Protein	Carbs	Fat	
Breakfast Totals							

SNACK	Time:	Amount	Calories	Protein	Carbs	Fat	
Snack Totals							

LUNCH	Time:	Amount	Calories	Protein	Carbs	Fat	
Lunch Totals							

SNACK	Time:	Amount	Calories	Protein	Carbs	Fat	
Snack Totals							

DINNER	Time:	Amount	Calories	Protein	Carbs	Fat	
Dinner Totals							

SNACK	Time:	Amount	Calories	Protein	Carbs	Fat	
Snack Totals							
DAY'S TOTALS							

Water Intake (8-oz servings)

Fruit/Vegetable Servings

Physical Activity	Duration	Calories Burned
Total Calories Burned		

Rate Your Day

1 2 3 4 5
6 7 8 9 10

Well Done

Keep Trying

DATE: / /

Mon ○ Tue ● Wed
○ Thu ● Fri ○ Sat ○ Sun

BREAKFAST	Time:	Amount	Calories	Protein	Carbs	Fat	
Breakfast Totals							

SNACK	Time:	Amount	Calories	Protein	Carbs	Fat	
Snack Totals							

LUNCH	Time:	Amount	Calories	Protein	Carbs	Fat	
Lunch Totals							

SNACK	Time:	Amount	Calories	Protein	Carbs	Fat	
Snack Totals							

DINNER	Time:	Amount	Calories	Protein	Carbs	Fat	
Dinner Totals							

SNACK	Time:	Amount	Calories	Protein	Carbs	Fat	
Snack Totals							
DAY'S TOTALS							

Water Intake (8-oz servings)

Fruit/Vegetable Servings

Physical Activity	Duration	Calories Burned
Total Calories Burned		

Rate Your Day

1 2 3 4 5
6 7 8 9 10

Well Done

Keep Trying

DATE: / /

BREAKFAST	Time:	Amount	Calories	Protein	Carbs	Fat	
Breakfast Totals							

SNACK	Time:	Amount	Calories	Protein	Carbs	Fat	
Snack Totals							

LUNCH	Time:	Amount	Calories	Protein	Carbs	Fat	
Lunch Totals							

SNACK	Time:	Amount	Calories	Protein	Carbs	Fat	
Snack Totals							

DINNER	Time:	Amount	Calories	Protein	Carbs	Fat	
Dinner Totals							

SNACK	Time:	Amount	Calories	Protein	Carbs	Fat	
Snack Totals							
DAY'S TOTALS							

Water Intake (8-oz servings)

Fruit/Vegetable Servings

Physical Activity	Duration	Calories Burned
Total Calories Burned		

Rate Your Day

1 2 3 4 5
6 7 8 9 10

Well Done

Keep Trying

DATE: / /

Mon ● Tue ● Wed ●
Thu ● Fri ● Sat ● Sun ●

BREAKFAST Time:	Amount	Calories	Protein	Carbs	Fat	
Breakfast Totals						

SNACK Time:	Amount	Calories	Protein	Carbs	Fat	
Snack Totals						

LUNCH Time:	Amount	Calories	Protein	Carbs	Fat	
Lunch Totals						

SNACK Time:	Amount	Calories	Protein	Carbs	Fat	
Snack Totals						

MY FOOD JOURNAL

DINNER	Time:	Amount	Calories	Protein	Carbs	Fat	
Dinner Totals							

SNACK	Time:	Amount	Calories	Protein	Carbs	Fat	
Snack Totals							
DAY'S TOTALS							

Water Intake (8-oz servings)

Fruit/Vegetable Servings

Physical Activity	Duration	Calories Burned
Total Calories Burned		

Rate Your Day

1 2 3 4 5
6 7 8 9 10

Well Done

Keep Trying

DATE: / /

○ Mon ○ Tue ● Wed
○ Thu ○ Fri ○ Sat ○ Sun

BREAKFAST	Time:	Amount	Calories	Protein	Carbs	Fat	
Breakfast Totals							

SNACK	Time:	Amount	Calories	Protein	Carbs	Fat	
Snack Totals							

LUNCH	Time:	Amount	Calories	Protein	Carbs	Fat	
Lunch Totals							

SNACK	Time:	Amount	Calories	Protein	Carbs	Fat	
Snack Totals							

DINNER	Time:	Amount	Calories	Protein	Carbs	Fat	
Dinner Totals							

SNACK	Time:	Amount	Calories	Protein	Carbs	Fat	
Snack Totals							
DAY'S TOTALS							

Water Intake (8-oz servings)

Fruit/Vegetable Servings

Physical Activity	Duration	Calories Burned
Total Calories Burned		

Rate Your Day

1 2 3 4 5
6 7 8 9 10

Well Done

Keep Trying

DATE: / /

Mon Tue **Wed**
Thu Fri Sat Sun

BREAKFAST	Time:	Amount	Calories	Protein	Carbs	Fat	
Breakfast Totals							

SNACK	Time:	Amount	Calories	Protein	Carbs	Fat	
Snack Totals							

LUNCH	Time:	Amount	Calories	Protein	Carbs	Fat	
Lunch Totals							

SNACK	Time:	Amount	Calories	Protein	Carbs	Fat	
Snack Totals							

DINNER	Time:	Amount	Calories	Protein	Carbs	Fat	
Dinner Totals							

SNACK	Time:	Amount	Calories	Protein	Carbs	Fat	
Snack Totals							
DAY'S TOTALS							

Water Intake (8-oz servings)

Fruit/Vegetable Servings

Physical Activity		Duration		Calories Burned
Total Calories Burned				

Rate Your Day

1 2 3 4 5
6 7 8 9 10

Well Done

Keep Trying

DATE: / /

○ Mon ○ Tue ● Wed
○ Thu ○ Fri ○ Sat ○ Sun

BREAKFAST Time:	Amount	Calories	Protein	Carbs	Fat	
Breakfast Totals						

SNACK Time:	Amount	Calories	Protein	Carbs	Fat	
Snack Totals						

LUNCH Time:	Amount	Calories	Protein	Carbs	Fat	
Lunch Totals						

SNACK Time:	Amount	Calories	Protein	Carbs	Fat	
Snack Totals						

DINNER	Time:	Amount	Calories	Protein	Carbs	Fat	
Dinner Totals							

SNACK	Time:	Amount	Calories	Protein	Carbs	Fat	
Snack Totals							
DAY'S TOTALS							

Water Intake (8-oz servings)

Fruit/Vegetable Servings

Physical Activity	Duration	Calories Burned
Total Calories Burned		

Rate Your Day

1 2 3 4 5
6 7 8 9 10

Well Done

Keep Trying

DATE: / /

Mon Tue **Wed**

Thu Fri Sat Sun

BREAKFAST	Time:	Amount	Calories	Protein	Carbs	Fat	
Breakfast Totals							

SNACK	Time:	Amount	Calories	Protein	Carbs	Fat	
Snack Totals							

LUNCH	Time:	Amount	Calories	Protein	Carbs	Fat	
Lunch Totals							

SNACK	Time:	Amount	Calories	Protein	Carbs	Fat	
Snack Totals							

DINNER	Time:	Amount	Calories	Protein	Carbs	Fat	
Dinner Totals							

SNACK	Time:	Amount	Calories	Protein	Carbs	Fat	
Snack Totals							
DAY'S TOTALS							

Water Intake (8-oz servings)

Fruit/Vegetable Servings

Physical Activity	Duration	Calories Burned
Total Calories Burned		

Rate Your Day

1 2 3 4 5
6 7 8 9 10

Well Done

Keep Trying

DATE: / /

Mon ● Tue ● **Wed**
Thu ● Fri ● Sat ● Sun

BREAKFAST	Time:	Amount	Calories	Protein	Carbs	Fat	
Breakfast Totals							

SNACK	Time:	Amount	Calories	Protein	Carbs	Fat	
Snack Totals							

LUNCH	Time:	Amount	Calories	Protein	Carbs	Fat	
Lunch Totals							

SNACK	Time:	Amount	Calories	Protein	Carbs	Fat	
Snack Totals							

MY FOOD JOURNAL

DINNER	Time:	Amount	Calories	Protein	Carbs	Fat	
Dinner Totals							

SNACK	Time:	Amount	Calories	Protein	Carbs	Fat	
Snack Totals							
DAY'S TOTALS							

Water Intake (8-oz servings)

Fruit/Vegetable Servings

Physical Activity	Duration	Calories Burned
Total Calories Burned		

Rate Your Day

1 2 3 4 5
6 7 8 9 10

Well Done

Keep Trying

DATE: / /

Mon ● Tue ● Wed ●
Thu ● Fri ● Sat ● Sun ●

BREAKFAST	Time:	Amount	Calories	Protein	Carbs	Fat	
Breakfast Totals							

SNACK	Time:	Amount	Calories	Protein	Carbs	Fat	
Snack Totals							

LUNCH	Time:	Amount	Calories	Protein	Carbs	Fat	
Lunch Totals							

SNACK	Time:	Amount	Calories	Protein	Carbs	Fat	
Snack Totals							

MY FOOD JOURNAL

DINNER	Time:	Amount	Calories	Protein	Carbs	Fat	
Dinner Totals							

SNACK	Time:	Amount	Calories	Protein	Carbs	Fat	
Snack Totals							
DAY'S TOTALS							

Water Intake (8-oz servings)

Fruit/Vegetable Servings

Physical Activity	Duration	Calories Burned
Total Calories Burned		

Rate Your Day

1 2 3 4 5
6 7 8 9 10

Well Done

Keep Trying

DATE: / /

Mon ● Tue ● **Wed** ● Thu ● Fri ● Sat ● Sun

BREAKFAST Time:	Amount	Calories	Protein	Carbs	Fat	
Breakfast Totals						

SNACK Time:	Amount	Calories	Protein	Carbs	Fat	
Snack Totals						

LUNCH Time:	Amount	Calories	Protein	Carbs	Fat	
Lunch Totals						

SNACK Time:	Amount	Calories	Protein	Carbs	Fat	
Snack Totals						

DINNER	Time:	Amount	Calories	Protein	Carbs	Fat	
Dinner Totals							

SNACK	Time:	Amount	Calories	Protein	Carbs	Fat	
Snack Totals							
DAY'S TOTALS							

Water Intake (8-oz servings)

Fruit/Vegetable Servings

Physical Activity	Duration	Calories Burned
Total Calories Burned		

Rate Your Day

① ② ③ ④ ⑤
⑥ ⑦ ⑧ ⑨ ⑩

Well Done

Keep Trying

DATE: / /

Mon ● Tue ● **Wed**
Thu ● Fri ● Sat ● Sun

BREAKFAST	Time:	Amount	Calories	Protein	Carbs	Fat	
Breakfast Totals							

SNACK	Time:	Amount	Calories	Protein	Carbs	Fat	
Snack Totals							

LUNCH	Time:	Amount	Calories	Protein	Carbs	Fat	
Lunch Totals							

SNACK	Time:	Amount	Calories	Protein	Carbs	Fat	
Snack Totals							

DINNER	Time:	Amount	Calories	Protein	Carbs	Fat	
Dinner Totals							

SNACK	Time:	Amount	Calories	Protein	Carbs	Fat	
Snack Totals							
DAY'S TOTALS							

Water Intake (8-oz servings)

Fruit/Vegetable Servings

Physical Activity	Duration	Calories Burned
Total Calories Burned		

Rate Your Day

1 2 3 4 5
6 7 8 9 10

Well Done

Keep Trying

DATE: / /

BREAKFAST	Time:	Amount	Calories	Protein	Carbs	Fat	
Breakfast Totals							

SNACK	Time:	Amount	Calories	Protein	Carbs	Fat	
Snack Totals							

LUNCH	Time:	Amount	Calories	Protein	Carbs	Fat	
Lunch Totals							

SNACK	Time:	Amount	Calories	Protein	Carbs	Fat	
Snack Totals							

DINNER	Time:	Amount	Calories	Protein	Carbs	Fat	
Dinner Totals							

SNACK	Time:	Amount	Calories	Protein	Carbs	Fat	
Snack Totals							
DAY'S TOTALS							

Water Intake (8-oz servings)

Fruit/Vegetable Servings

Physical Activity	Duration	Calories Burned
Total Calories Burned		

Rate Your Day

1 2 3 4 5
6 7 8 9 10

Well Done

Keep Trying

DATE: / /

Mon ● Tue ○ Wed ●
Thu ○ Fri ● Sat ○ Sun ○

BREAKFAST	Time:	Amount	Calories	Protein	Carbs	Fat	
Breakfast Totals							

SNACK	Time:	Amount	Calories	Protein	Carbs	Fat	
Snack Totals							

LUNCH	Time:	Amount	Calories	Protein	Carbs	Fat	
Lunch Totals							

SNACK	Time:	Amount	Calories	Protein	Carbs	Fat	
Snack Totals							

DINNER	Time:	Amount	Calories	Protein	Carbs	Fat	
Dinner Totals							

SNACK	Time:	Amount	Calories	Protein	Carbs	Fat	
Snack Totals							
DAY'S TOTALS							

Water Intake (8-oz servings)

Fruit/Vegetable Servings

Physical Activity	Duration	Calories Burned
Total Calories Burned		

Rate Your Day

1 2 3 4 5
6 7 8 9 10

Well Done

Keep Trying

DATE: / /

○ Mon ○ Tue ● Wed
○ Thu ○ Fri ○ Sat ○ Sun

BREAKFAST	Time:	Amount	Calories	Protein	Carbs	Fat	
Breakfast Totals							

SNACK	Time:	Amount	Calories	Protein	Carbs	Fat	
Snack Totals							

LUNCH	Time:	Amount	Calories	Protein	Carbs	Fat	
Lunch Totals							

SNACK	Time:	Amount	Calories	Protein	Carbs	Fat	
Snack Totals							

DINNER	Time:	Amount	Calories	Protein	Carbs	Fat	
Dinner Totals							

SNACK	Time:	Amount	Calories	Protein	Carbs	Fat	
Snack Totals							
DAY'S TOTALS							

Water Intake (8-oz servings)

Fruit/Vegetable Servings

Physical Activity	Duration	Calories Burned
Total Calories Burned		

Rate Your Day

1 2 3 4 5
6 7 8 9 10

Well Done

Keep Trying

DATE: / /

Mon Tue ●Wed
Thu ●Fri Sat Sun

BREAKFAST Time:	Amount	Calories	Protein	Carbs	Fat	
Breakfast Totals						

SNACK Time:	Amount	Calories	Protein	Carbs	Fat	
Snack Totals						

LUNCH Time:	Amount	Calories	Protein	Carbs	Fat	
Lunch Totals						

SNACK Time:	Amount	Calories	Protein	Carbs	Fat	
Snack Totals						

DINNER	Time:	Amount	Calories	Protein	Carbs	Fat	
Dinner Totals							

SNACK	Time:	Amount	Calories	Protein	Carbs	Fat	
Snack Totals							
DAY'S TOTALS							

Water Intake (8-oz servings)

Fruit/Vegetable Servings

Physical Activity	Duration	Calories Burned
Total Calories Burned		

Rate Your Day

1 2 3 4 5
6 7 8 9 10

Well Done	Keep Trying

DATE: / /

Mon ● Tue ● **Wed**
Thu ● Fri ● Sat ● Sun

BREAKFAST	Time:	Amount	Calories	Protein	Carbs	Fat	
Breakfast Totals							

SNACK	Time:	Amount	Calories	Protein	Carbs	Fat	
Snack Totals							

LUNCH	Time:	Amount	Calories	Protein	Carbs	Fat	
Lunch Totals							

SNACK	Time:	Amount	Calories	Protein	Carbs	Fat	
Snack Totals							

DINNER	Time:	Amount	Calories	Protein	Carbs	Fat	
Dinner Totals							

SNACK	Time:	Amount	Calories	Protein	Carbs	Fat	
Snack Totals							
DAY'S TOTALS							

Water Intake (8-oz servings)

Fruit/Vegetable Servings

Physical Activity	Duration	Calories Burned
Total Calories Burned		

Rate Your Day

1 2 3 4 5
6 7 8 9 10

Well Done

Keep Trying

DATE: / /

BREAKFAST	Time:	Amount	Calories	Protein	Carbs	Fat	
Breakfast Totals							

SNACK	Time:	Amount	Calories	Protein	Carbs	Fat	
Snack Totals							

LUNCH	Time:	Amount	Calories	Protein	Carbs	Fat	
Lunch Totals							

SNACK	Time:	Amount	Calories	Protein	Carbs	Fat	
Snack Totals							

DINNER	Time:	Amount	Calories	Protein	Carbs	Fat	
Dinner Totals							

SNACK	Time:	Amount	Calories	Protein	Carbs	Fat	
Snack Totals							
DAY'S TOTALS							

Water Intake (8-oz servings)

Fruit/Vegetable Servings

Physical Activity	Duration	Calories Burned
Total Calories Burned		

Rate Your Day

1 2 3 4 5
6 7 8 9 10

Well Done

Keep Trying

DATE: / /

○ Mon ○ Tue ● Wed
○ Thu ○ Fri ○ Sat ○ Sun

BREAKFAST	Time:	Amount	Calories	Protein	Carbs	Fat	
Breakfast Totals							

SNACK	Time:	Amount	Calories	Protein	Carbs	Fat	
Snack Totals							

LUNCH	Time:	Amount	Calories	Protein	Carbs	Fat	
Lunch Totals							

SNACK	Time:	Amount	Calories	Protein	Carbs	Fat	
Snack Totals							

DINNER	Time:	Amount	Calories	Protein	Carbs	Fat	
Dinner Totals							

SNACK	Time:	Amount	Calories	Protein	Carbs	Fat	
Snack Totals							
DAY'S TOTALS							

Water Intake (8-oz servings)

Fruit/Vegetable Servings

Physical Activity	Duration	Calories Burned
Total Calories Burned		

Rate Your Day

1 2 3 4 5
6 7 8 9 10

Well Done

Keep Trying

DATE: / /

Mon ◯ Tue ● Wed
◯ Thu ● Fri ◯ Sat ◯ Sun

BREAKFAST	Time:	Amount	Calories	Protein	Carbs	Fat	
Breakfast Totals							

SNACK	Time:	Amount	Calories	Protein	Carbs	Fat	
Snack Totals							

LUNCH	Time:	Amount	Calories	Protein	Carbs	Fat	
Lunch Totals		.					

SNACK	Time:	Amount	Calories	Protein	Carbs	Fat	
Snack Totals							

DINNER	Time:	Amount	Calories	Protein	Carbs	Fat	
Dinner Totals							

SNACK	Time:	Amount	Calories	Protein	Carbs	Fat	
Snack Totals							
DAY'S TOTALS							

Water Intake (8-oz servings)

Fruit/Vegetable Servings

Physical Activity	Duration	Calories Burned
Total Calories Burned		

Rate Your Day

1 2 3 4 5
6 7 8 9 10

Well Done

Keep Trying

DATE: / /

Mon ○ Tue ● Wed
○ Thu ○ Fri ○ Sat ○ Sun

BREAKFAST	Time:	Amount	Calories	Protein	Carbs	Fat	
Breakfast Totals							

SNACK	Time:	Amount	Calories	Protein	Carbs	Fat	
Snack Totals							

LUNCH	Time:	Amount	Calories	Protein	Carbs	Fat	
Lunch Totals							

SNACK	Time:	Amount	Calories	Protein	Carbs	Fat	
Snack Totals							

DINNER	Time:	Amount	Calories	Protein	Carbs	Fat	
Dinner Totals							

SNACK	Time:	Amount	Calories	Protein	Carbs	Fat	
Snack Totals							
DAY'S TOTALS							

Water Intake (8-oz servings)

Fruit/Vegetable Servings

Physical Activity	Duration	Calories Burned
Total Calories Burned		

Rate Your Day

1 2 3 4 5
6 7 8 9 10

Well Done

Keep Trying

DATE: / /

BREAKFAST	Time:	Amount	Calories	Protein	Carbs	Fat	
Breakfast Totals							

SNACK	Time:	Amount	Calories	Protein	Carbs	Fat	
Snack Totals							

LUNCH	Time:	Amount	Calories	Protein	Carbs	Fat	
Lunch Totals							

SNACK	Time:	Amount	Calories	Protein	Carbs	Fat	
Snack Totals							

DINNER	Time:	Amount	Calories	Protein	Carbs	Fat	
Dinner Totals							

SNACK	Time:	Amount	Calories	Protein	Carbs	Fat	
Snack Totals							
DAY'S TOTALS							

Water Intake (8-oz servings)

Fruit/Vegetable Servings

Physical Activity	Duration	Calories Burned
Total Calories Burned		

Rate Your Day

1 2 3 4 5
6 7 8 9 10

Well Done

Keep Trying

DATE: / /

Mon ● Tue ● **Wed** ●
Thu ● Fri ● Sat ● Sun ●

BREAKFAST	Time:	Amount	Calories	Protein	Carbs	Fat	
Breakfast Totals							

SNACK	Time:	Amount	Calories	Protein	Carbs	Fat	
Snack Totals							

LUNCH	Time:	Amount	Calories	Protein	Carbs	Fat	
Lunch Totals							

SNACK	Time:	Amount	Calories	Protein	Carbs	Fat	
Snack Totals							

DINNER	Time:	Amount	Calories	Protein	Carbs	Fat	
Dinner Totals							

SNACK	Time:	Amount	Calories	Protein	Carbs	Fat	
Snack Totals							
DAY'S TOTALS							

Water Intake (8-oz servings)

Fruit/Vegetable Servings

Physical Activity	Duration	Calories Burned
Total Calories Burned		

Rate Your Day

① ② ③ ④ ⑤
⑥ ⑦ ⑧ ⑨ ⑩

Well Done

Keep Trying

DATE: / /

BREAKFAST	Time:	Amount	Calories	Protein	Carbs	Fat	
Breakfast Totals							

SNACK	Time:	Amount	Calories	Protein	Carbs	Fat	
Snack Totals							

LUNCH	Time:	Amount	Calories	Protein	Carbs	Fat	
Lunch Totals							

SNACK	Time:	Amount	Calories	Protein	Carbs	Fat	
Snack Totals							

DINNER	Time:	Amount	Calories	Protein	Carbs	Fat	
Dinner Totals							

SNACK	Time:	Amount	Calories	Protein	Carbs	Fat	
Snack Totals							
DAY'S TOTALS							

Water Intake (8-oz servings)

Fruit/Vegetable Servings

Physical Activity	Duration	Calories Burned
Total Calories Burned		

Rate Your Day

1 2 3 4 5
6 7 8 9 10

Well Done

Keep Trying

DATE: / /

Mon Tue **Wed**
Thu Fri Sat Sun

BREAKFAST	Time:	Amount	Calories	Protein	Carbs	Fat	
Breakfast Totals							

SNACK	Time:	Amount	Calories	Protein	Carbs	Fat	
Snack Totals							

LUNCH	Time:	Amount	Calories	Protein	Carbs	Fat	
Lunch Totals							

SNACK	Time:	Amount	Calories	Protein	Carbs	Fat	
Snack Totals							

DINNER	Time:	Amount	Calories	Protein	Carbs	Fat	
Dinner Totals							

SNACK	Time:	Amount	Calories	Protein	Carbs	Fat	
Snack Totals							
DAY'S TOTALS							

Water Intake (8-oz servings)

Fruit/Vegetable Servings

Physical Activity	Duration	Calories Burned
Total Calories Burned		

Rate Your Day

1 2 3 4 5
6 7 8 9 10

Well Done

Keep Trying

DATE: / /

Mon Tue **Wed**
Thu Fri Sat Sun

BREAKFAST	Time:	Amount	Calories	Protein	Carbs	Fat	
Breakfast Totals							

SNACK	Time:	Amount	Calories	Protein	Carbs	Fat	
Snack Totals							

LUNCH	Time:	Amount	Calories	Protein	Carbs	Fat	
Lunch Totals							

SNACK	Time:	Amount	Calories	Protein	Carbs	Fat	
Snack Totals							

DINNER	Time:	Amount	Calories	Protein	Carbs	Fat	
Dinner Totals							

SNACK	Time:	Amount	Calories	Protein	Carbs	Fat	
Snack Totals							
DAY'S TOTALS							

Water Intake (8-oz servings)

Fruit/Vegetable Servings

Physical Activity	Duration	Calories Burned
Total Calories Burned		

Rate Your Day

1 2 3 4 5
6 7 8 9 10

Well Done

Keep Trying

DATE: / /

Mon Tue **Wed**
Thu Fri Sat Sun

BREAKFAST Time:	Amount	Calories	Protein	Carbs	Fat	
Breakfast Totals						

SNACK Time:	Amount	Calories	Protein	Carbs	Fat	
Snack Totals						

LUNCH Time:	Amount	Calories	Protein	Carbs	Fat	
Lunch Totals						

SNACK Time:	Amount	Calories	Protein	Carbs	Fat	
Snack Totals						

DINNER	Time:	Amount	Calories	Protein	Carbs	Fat	
Dinner Totals							

SNACK	Time:	Amount	Calories	Protein	Carbs	Fat	
Snack Totals							
DAY'S TOTALS							

Water Intake (8-oz servings)

Fruit/Vegetable Servings

Physical Activity	Duration	Calories Burned
Total Calories Burned		

Rate Your Day

1 2 3 4 5
6 7 8 9 10

Well Done

Keep Trying

DATE: / /

Mon ◯ Tue ◯ Wed ⬤
Thu ◯ Fri ⬤ Sat ◯ Sun ◯

BREAKFAST	Time:	Amount	Calories	Protein	Carbs	Fat	
Breakfast Totals							

SNACK	Time:	Amount	Calories	Protein	Carbs	Fat	
Snack Totals							

LUNCH	Time:	Amount	Calories	Protein	Carbs	Fat	
Lunch Totals							

SNACK	Time:	Amount	Calories	Protein	Carbs	Fat	
Snack Totals							

DINNER	Time:	Amount	Calories	Protein	Carbs	Fat	
Dinner Totals							

SNACK	Time:	Amount	Calories	Protein	Carbs	Fat	
Snack Totals							
DAY'S TOTALS							

Water Intake (8-oz servings)

Fruit/Vegetable Servings

Physical Activity	Duration	Calories Burned
Total Calories Burned		

Rate Your Day

1 2 3 4 5
6 7 8 9 10

Well Done

Keep Trying

DATE: / /

BREAKFAST	Time:	Amount	Calories	Protein	Carbs	Fat	
Breakfast Totals							

SNACK	Time:	Amount	Calories	Protein	Carbs	Fat	
Snack Totals							

LUNCH	Time:	Amount	Calories	Protein	Carbs	Fat	
Lunch Totals							

SNACK	Time:	Amount	Calories	Protein	Carbs	Fat	
Snack Totals							

DINNER	Time:	Amount	Calories	Protein	Carbs	Fat	
Dinner Totals							

SNACK	Time:	Amount	Calories	Protein	Carbs	Fat	
Snack Totals							
DAY'S TOTALS							

Water Intake (8-oz servings)

Fruit/Vegetable Servings

Physical Activity	Duration	Calories Burned
Total Calories Burned		

Rate Your Day

1 2 3 4 5
6 7 8 9 10

Well Done

Keep Trying

DATE: / /

Mon ○ Tue ● Wed ○
Thu ○ Fri ○ Sat ○ Sun ○

BREAKFAST Time:	Amount	Calories	Protein	Carbs	Fat	
Breakfast Totals						

SNACK Time:	Amount	Calories	Protein	Carbs	Fat	
Snack Totals						

LUNCH Time:	Amount	Calories	Protein	Carbs	Fat	
Lunch Totals						

SNACK Time:	Amount	Calories	Protein	Carbs	Fat	
Snack Totals						

DINNER	Time:	Amount	Calories	Protein	Carbs	Fat	
Dinner Totals							

SNACK	Time:	Amount	Calories	Protein	Carbs	Fat	
Snack Totals							
DAY'S TOTALS							

Water Intake (8-oz servings)

Fruit/Vegetable Servings

Physical Activity	Duration	Calories Burned
Total Calories Burned		

Rate Your Day

1 2 3 4 5
6 7 8 9 10

Well Done

Keep Trying

DATE: / /

Mon Tue ● Wed
Thu Fri Sat Sun

BREAKFAST Time:	Amount	Calories	Protein	Carbs	Fat	
Breakfast Totals						

SNACK Time:	Amount	Calories	Protein	Carbs	Fat	
Snack Totals						

LUNCH Time:	Amount	Calories	Protein	Carbs	Fat	
Lunch Totals						

SNACK Time:	Amount	Calories	Protein	Carbs	Fat	
Snack Totals						

DINNER	Time:	Amount	Calories	Protein	Carbs	Fat	
Dinner Totals							

SNACK	Time:	Amount	Calories	Protein	Carbs	Fat	
Snack Totals							
DAY'S TOTALS							

Water Intake (8-oz servings)

Fruit/Vegetable Servings

Physical Activity	Duration	Calories Burned
Total Calories Burned		

Rate Your Day

1 2 3 4 5
6 7 8 9 10

Well Done

Keep Trying

DATE: / /

Mon ● Tue ● Wed
Thu ● Fri ● Sat ● Sun

BREAKFAST	Time:	Amount	Calories	Protein	Carbs	Fat	
Breakfast Totals							

SNACK	Time:	Amount	Calories	Protein	Carbs	Fat	
Snack Totals							

LUNCH	Time:	Amount	Calories	Protein	Carbs	Fat	
Lunch Totals							

SNACK	Time:	Amount	Calories	Protein	Carbs	Fat	
Snack Totals							

DINNER	Time:	Amount	Calories	Protein	Carbs	Fat	
Dinner Totals							

SNACK	Time:	Amount	Calories	Protein	Carbs	Fat	
Snack Totals							
DAY'S TOTALS							

Water Intake (8-oz servings)

Fruit/Vegetable Servings

Physical Activity	Duration	Calories Burned
Total Calories Burned		

Rate Your Day

1 2 3 4 5
6 7 8 9 10

Well Done

Keep Trying

DATE: / /

○ Mon ○ Tue ● Wed
○ Thu ○ Fri ○ Sat ○ Sun

BREAKFAST Time:	Amount	Calories	Protein	Carbs	Fat	
Breakfast Totals						

SNACK Time:	Amount	Calories	Protein	Carbs	Fat	
Snack Totals						

LUNCH Time:	Amount	Calories	Protein	Carbs	Fat	
Lunch Totals						

SNACK Time:	Amount	Calories	Protein	Carbs	Fat	
Snack Totals						

DINNER	Time:	Amount	Calories	Protein	Carbs	Fat	
Dinner Totals							

SNACK	Time:	Amount	Calories	Protein	Carbs	Fat	
Snack Totals							
DAY'S TOTALS							

Water Intake (8-oz servings)

Fruit/Vegetable Servings

Physical Activity	Duration	Calories Burned
Total Calories Burned		

Rate Your Day

1 2 3 4 5
6 7 8 9 10

Well Done

Keep Trying

DATE: / /

Mon Tue **Wed**
Thu Fri Sat Sun

BREAKFAST	Time:	Amount	Calories	Protein	Carbs	Fat	
Breakfast Totals							

SNACK	Time:	Amount	Calories	Protein	Carbs	Fat	
Snack Totals							

LUNCH	Time:	Amount	Calories	Protein	Carbs	Fat	
Lunch Totals							

SNACK	Time:	Amount	Calories	Protein	Carbs	Fat	
Snack Totals							

DINNER	Time:	Amount	Calories	Protein	Carbs	Fat	
Dinner Totals							

SNACK	Time:	Amount	Calories	Protein	Carbs	Fat	
Snack Totals							
DAY'S TOTALS							

Water Intake (8-oz servings)

Fruit/Vegetable Servings

Physical Activity	Duration	Calories Burned
Total Calories Burned		

Rate Your Day

1 2 3 4 5
6 7 8 9 10

Well Done

Keep Trying

DATE: / /

○ Mon ○ Tue ● Wed
○ Thu ○ Fri ○ Sat ○ Sun

BREAKFAST Time:	Amount	Calories	Protein	Carbs	Fat	
Breakfast Totals						

SNACK Time:	Amount	Calories	Protein	Carbs	Fat	
Snack Totals						

LUNCH Time:	Amount	Calories	Protein	Carbs	Fat	
Lunch Totals						

SNACK Time:	Amount	Calories	Protein	Carbs	Fat	
Snack Totals						

DINNER	Time:	Amount	Calories	Protein	Carbs	Fat	
Dinner Totals							

SNACK	Time:	Amount	Calories	Protein	Carbs	Fat	
Snack Totals							
DAY'S TOTALS							

Water Intake (8-oz servings)

Fruit/Vegetable Servings

Physical Activity	Duration	Calories Burned
Total Calories Burned		

Rate Your Day

1 2 3 4 5
6 7 8 9 10

Well Done

Keep Trying

DATE: / /

● Mon ● Tue ● Wed
● Thu ● Fri ● Sat ● Sun

BREAKFAST	Time:	Amount	Calories	Protein	Carbs	Fat	
Breakfast Totals							

SNACK	Time:	Amount	Calories	Protein	Carbs	Fat	
Snack Totals							

LUNCH	Time:	Amount	Calories	Protein	Carbs	Fat	
Lunch Totals							

SNACK	Time:	Amount	Calories	Protein	Carbs	Fat	
Snack Totals							

DINNER	Time:	Amount	Calories	Protein	Carbs	Fat	
Dinner Totals							

SNACK	Time:	Amount	Calories	Protein	Carbs	Fat	
Snack Totals							
DAY'S TOTALS							

Water Intake (8-oz servings)

Fruit/Vegetable Servings

Physical Activity	Duration	Calories Burned
Total Calories Burned		

Rate Your Day

1 2 3 4 5
6 7 8 9 10

Well Done

Keep Trying

DATE: / /

○ Mon ○ Tue ● Wed
○ Thu ○ Fri ○ Sat ○ Sun

BREAKFAST Time:	Amount	Calories	Protein	Carbs	Fat	
Breakfast Totals						

SNACK Time:	Amount	Calories	Protein	Carbs	Fat	
Snack Totals						

LUNCH Time:	Amount	Calories	Protein	Carbs	Fat	
Lunch Totals						

SNACK Time:	Amount	Calories	Protein	Carbs	Fat	
Snack Totals						

DINNER	Time:	Amount	Calories	Protein	Carbs	Fat	
Dinner Totals							

SNACK	Time:	Amount	Calories	Protein	Carbs	Fat	
Snack Totals							
DAY'S TOTALS							

Water Intake (8-oz servings)

Fruit/Vegetable Servings

Physical Activity	Duration	Calories Burned
Total Calories Burned		

Rate Your Day

1 2 3 4 5
6 7 8 9 10

Well Done

Keep Trying

Today I celebrate this progress from the first day I began journaling:

I'm also proud of these little victories along the way:

What I've learned about myself and my habits through my journaling:

My next goals and action steps toward them: